ESOPHAGEAL CANCER

Current and Emerging Trends in Detection and Treatment

JANEY LEVY

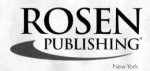

ROSEN
PUBLISHING®
New York

Published in 2012 by The Rosen Publishing Group, Inc.
29 East 21st Street, New York, NY 10010

Library of Congress Cataloging-in-Publication Data

Levy, Janey.
Esophageal cancer: current and emerging trends in detection and treatment / Janey Levy.—1st ed.
    p. cm.—(Cancer and modern science)
Includes bibliographical references and index.
ISBN 978-1-4488-1310-0 (lib. bdg.)
1. Esophagus—Cancer—Juvenile literature. I. Title.
RC280.E8L48 2012
616.99'432—dc22

                                                                        2010011323

Manufactured in the United States of America

CPSIA Compliance Information: Batch #S11YA: For further information, contact Rosen Publishing, New York, New York, at 1-800-237-9932.

On the cover: This highly magnified image, taken through a microscope, provides a clear view of esophageal cancer cells. The cells have been stained purple to make structural details easier to see.

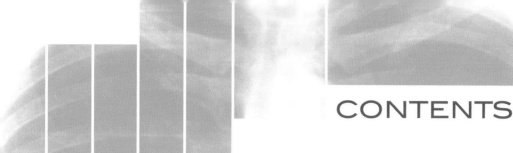

CONTENTS

INTRODUCTION

Almost everyone is familiar with cancer. The news frequently reports the deaths of famous people from cancer and the results of new cancer research. Cancer kills hundreds of thousands of people annually. In "The History of Cancer," the American Cancer Society (ACS) identifies cancer as the second-leading cause of death in the United States. The document also states that half of men and one-third of women in the United States will develop cancer during their lifetimes. Many individuals reading this may have family members or friends who have had cancer or may have had it themselves. Yet in spite of cancer's looming presence in today's world, how well do most people understand it? What exactly is cancer?

Cancer is a disease of the genes, the basic units of heredity that everyone carries in their cells. However, that statement is slightly misleading. Cancer isn't a single disease. It's many diseases that share common features. Cancer results from genetic mutations, or changes in genes. These mutations may result from environmental factors. They may be inherited. Sometimes, they have no clear cause.

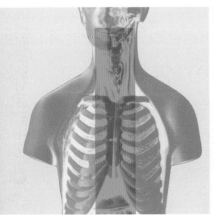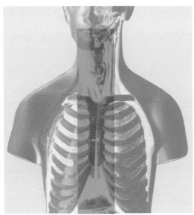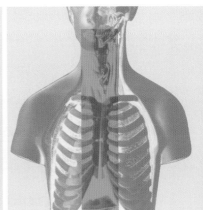

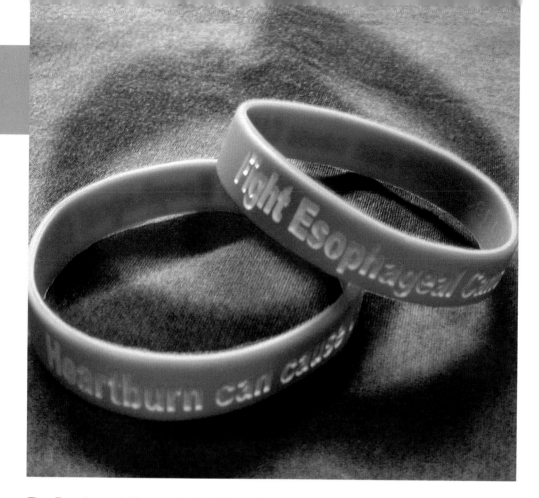

The Esophageal Cancer Action Network sells these periwinkle blue wristbands to promote awareness of the disease. One side reads "Fight Esophageal Cancer." The other reads "Heartburn can cause CANCER."

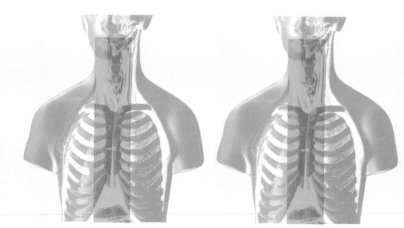

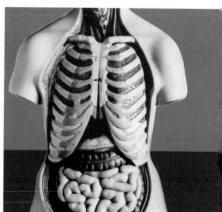

How do genetic mutations cause cancer? They allow cells to grow uncontrollably, which (usually) produces tumors. Although some tumors are benign, or harmless, others aren't. Malignant tumors seriously harm a person's health, may spread to other parts of the body, and may cause death. They are cancer.

Two familiar and common cancers are lung cancer and breast cancer. These cancers cause tens of thousands of deaths annually. Many millions of dollars have been spent on research to develop better methods of detecting and treating them. Yet these diseases are just the tip of the cancer iceberg. Cancer can occur just about anywhere in the body, including the esophagus.

The esophagus is the muscular tube that carries food and liquid from the mouth to the stomach. Two types of esophageal cancer exist: squamous cell carcinoma and adenocarcinoma. Unfortunately, both types usually aren't diagnosed until the cancer is very advanced, so the death rate is high. About 85 percent of patients die within five years of being diagnosed, according to the ACS guide *Esophageal Cancer*. To make matters worse, the number of new cases being diagnosed each year is increasing rapidly.

Given the high death rate, it's natural to wonder if esophageal cancer can be prevented. No guaranteed means of prevention currently exist. However, people can take steps to lower their risk. Researchers have identified several risk factors for esophageal cancer. Although some are inherited conditions over which a person has no control, others are factors an individual can do something about, such as smoking and drinking too much alcohol. Still others are medical conditions that can be treated and monitored by physicians. There's reason to believe in a brighter future. Researchers are seeking better ways to treat esophageal cancer, detect it early, and perhaps even prevent it.

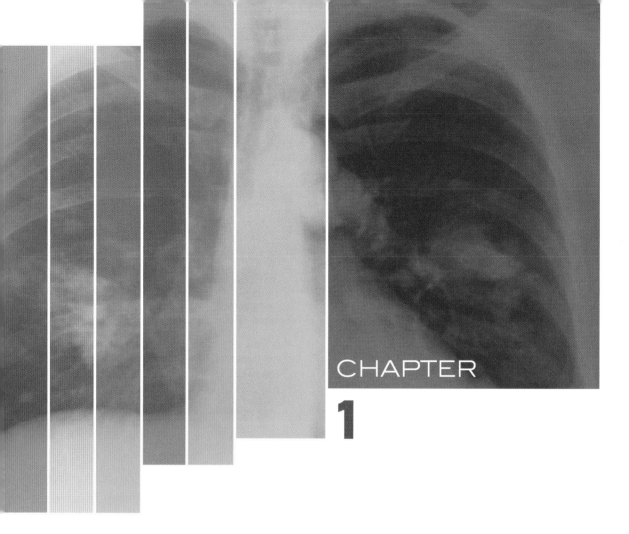

CHAPTER

1

DEVELOPMENTS IN THE SCIENCE OF ESOPHAGEAL CANCER THROUGHOUT HISTORY

Cancer is hardly a new disease. Humans have suffered from various forms of cancer throughout history. What is the evidence? For one thing, ancient remains showing signs of cancer have been discovered. The skull of a woman who lived almost four thousand years ago bears the oldest known specimen of human cancer. The record goes back much further. A jawbone from a human ancestor who lived 1.5 to 4 million years ago shows possible bone cancer.

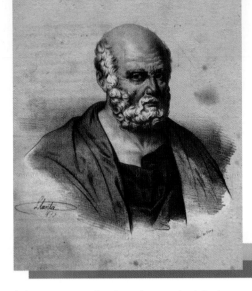

Cancer was well known to the ancient Greek physician Hippocrates, shown in this nineteenth-century portrait. Many modern cancer terms come from the writings of this great physician and his followers.

Ancient writings describing cancer also exist. An Egyptian papyrus created around 1600 BCE—likely a copy of one written around 3000 BCE—describes eight cases of what is probably breast cancer. Writings produced around 400 BCE by the great Greek physician Hippocrates and his followers contain many references to cancer. Roman writer Aulus Cornelius Celsus (25 BCE–50 CE) and Roman physician Claudius Galen (125–200 CE) also wrote about cancer.

Among these ancient texts, several describe what is probably esophageal cancer. The Egyptian papyrus is one example. There are also Chinese texts more than two thousand years old that contain accounts of esophageal cancer. Roman physician Galen wrote about fleshy growths that caused problems swallowing. In 1025, the great Islamic scientist Ibn Sīnā (known in Europe as Avicenna) wrote that difficulty swallowing was the primary symptom of esophageal tumors.

ANCIENT SCIENTIFIC THEORIES OF CANCER

Ancient civilizations developed their own theories about what causes cancer. Although these ideas differ greatly from modern scientific theories, they represent the scientific thought of their day. Ancient Egyptians, for instance, believed the gods caused cancer. Hippocrates believed cancer resulted from an imbalance of the four humors. The four humors were bodily fluids that were essential for a person's health—blood, phlegm, yellow bile, and black bile. When they were in proper balance, an individual was healthy. If they were unbalanced, illness resulted. In Hippocrates' view, an excess of black bile caused cancer. Galen accepted Hippocrates' ideas and repeated them in his own writings. His works were so influential that the theory of the four humors and how they influenced health lasted through the Renaissance.

WHERE "CANCER" AND RELATED TERMS COME FROM

The term "cancer" can be traced back to ancient Greece. Hippocrates (circa 460–370 BCE) and his followers used the words *karkinos* and *karkinoma* for tumors. These terms come from the word for "crab" and were probably chosen because the fingerlike projections radiating from a tumor resemble a crab. Roman writer Celsus translated *karkinos* into the Latin word for crab, *cancer*, establishing the term used today. The Greek *karkinoma* gave rise to "carcinoma," the modern term for cancers that originate in the epithelium, the tissue that lines the esophagus and other body parts. Instead of the terms favored by Hippocrates and his followers, Roman physician Galen used another Greek word—*onkos*, which means "mass" or "swelling." *Onkos* gave rise to the modern name for the medical field of cancer study—"oncology"—and the name for physicians in the field—"oncologists."

SCIENCE AND ESOPHAGEAL CANCER FROM THE RENAISSANCE TO 1900

Although Hippocrates' cancer theories remained influential, the Renaissance also saw the beginnings of modern scientific thought concerning esophageal cancer. For example, Andreas Vesalius, a young anatomist from what is today Belgium, provided knowledge of esophageal anatomy in a book published in 1543. Around the same time, French physician Jean François Fernel described esophageal tumors that caused problems in swallowing.

The texts of Vesalius and Fernel were standard medical writings—descriptions of what a scientist or physician observed in someone else's body. An extraordinary work of the late 1600s combined a scientist's powers of observation with the knowledge gained from personal experience. British surgeon John Casaubon, who died of esophageal cancer in 1691, left a written account of the symptoms he experienced.

During the 1700s, reports and descriptions of esophageal tumors increased. The earliest drawings of an esophageal tumor appeared in a book by Matthew Baillie published in 1799. Some understanding of the causes also emerged. For example, a 1770 article by E. G. Gyser linked heavy alcohol consumption to esophageal cancer.

The science of esophageal cancer expanded rapidly in the 1800s. German physician Phillip Bozzini invented the endoscope in 1806. This instrument allowed doctors to actually see into a living person's esophagus. British physician W. H. Walshe's 1846 description of esophageal cancer's rate of occurrence, site, form, type, symptoms, spread, and treatment reflected the enormous growth in knowledge of the disease.

Surgical treatment of esophageal cancer progressed after 1850. German surgeon Albrecht Theodor von Middeldorpf performed the first operation on an esophageal tumor in 1857. Another German surgeon, Theodor Billroth, practiced esophageal resections and reconnections on

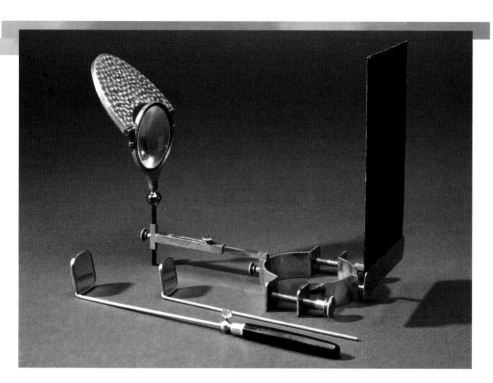

This was the late-nineteenth-century version of an endoscope. A physician stuck a long-handled small mirror down a patient's throat. A lens and mirror provided illumination by directing lamplight down the throat.

dogs in 1871. That is, he surgically removed part of the esophagus and then connected the remaining parts to each other. This paved the way for the procedure in humans. Billroth's son-in-law, Vincenz Czerny, performed the first successful resection of a human esophagus in 1877. Czerny suggested that cancer couldn't be controlled by surgery alone, and he developed ideas for combined treatments. An 1881 book by Scottish physician Alexander Monro provided what was probably the first description of the spread of cancer to and from the esophagus.

As a result of the work of these men and others, the twentieth century began with a much greater understanding of esophageal cancer than any previous century had possessed. Further advances came slowly, but the twentieth century saw the development of many new diagnostic and treatment tools.

SCIENCE AND ESOPHAGEAL CANCER SINCE 1900

Little development occurred in the first half of the twentieth century. However, physicians worked to refine endoscopes, and better endoscopes could improve diagnosis.

Early endoscopes were often rigid. This meant their use was difficult, painful for the patient, and potentially dangerous—they could easily puncture or tear the esophagus. The 1930s saw the development of semiflexible endoscopes. Nevertheless, it wasn't until the 1950s that dramatic advances were made.

In 1954, physician Basil Hirschowitz and two colleagues at the University of Michigan in Ann Arbor began work on a fiber-optic endoscope. Fiber-optic cable is a bundle of extremely thin glass or plastic fibers that transmits light and images. It permitted the creation of thin, flexible endoscopes. Hirschowitz finally had the kind of fiber-optic endoscope he wanted in 1957, and he tested it first on himself! This new instrument revolutionized endoscopy. It gave physicians a better view of the esophagus and made the procedure safer and more comfortable for patients. As a result, endoscopy became more common.

Other diagnostic advances include the identification in 1960 of Barrett's esophagus as a risk factor. New diagnostic tests—including barium swallows, CT scans, PET scans, and endoscopic ultrasound—appeared. These tests and others are described in chapter 4.

The late twentieth century also saw developments in treatment options. For most of the century, surgery had remained the standard treatment. New treatment options finally became available in the mid-1980s. These included radiation therapy, chemotherapy, and combination

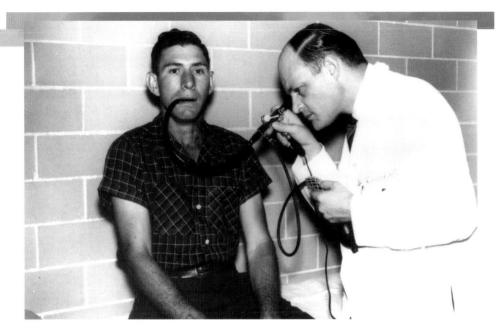

Shown here around 1960, Basil Hirschowitz demonstrates the fiber-optic endoscope he and two colleagues had recently developed. His original endoscope is now in the Smithsonian Institution in Washington, D.C.

therapy involving radiation therapy and chemotherapy together and/or combined with surgery. New "minimally invasive" surgical techniques were developed that required only tiny incisions. Endoscopic therapies appeared, too. These treatments are described along with diagnostic procedures in chapter 4.

The twentieth century saw a greatly increased understanding of what happens in esophageal and other cancers. This insight was largely due to advances in genetics, as the next chapter describes.

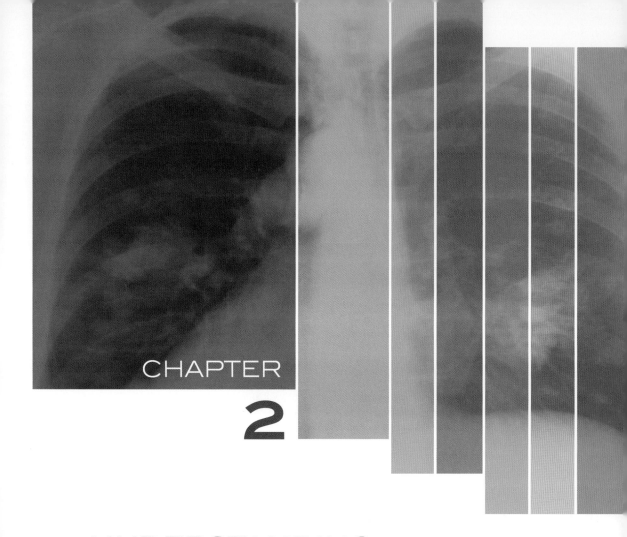

UNDERSTANDING WHAT HAPPENS IN ESOPHAGEAL CANCER

The esophagus is one of many organs that constitute the human body. Tissues make up the organs, and microscopic cells, invisible to the unaided eye, make up the tissues. The human body contains hundreds of millions of cells. The cell is where cancer begins.

Healthy cells in an individual's body don't live forever. Throughout a person's life, normal cells grow, divide to form new cells as the body needs them, and finally die. Cancer occurs when cells grow uncontrollably. This growth results from genetic mutations.

Genes and Mutations

Genes are the basic units of heredity. They carry information for such things as hair color, eye color, and height. They also determine whether a person will have or be prone to developing a genetic disease or disorder.

Genes

Genes are located on structures called chromosomes that are found in every cell in an organism. Chromosomes are composed of proteins and a substance called deoxyribonucleic acid, or DNA. An organism's complete set of DNA is its genome. Individual genes are stretches of DNA that tell the cell how to make the proteins necessary for life.

Chemical units called nucleotides make up DNA. Three nucleotides form a codon, and several codons form a gene. Each codon instructs the cell to make one of the amino acids that make up proteins. The sequence of nucleotides determines which amino acid is made. This sequence is the genetic code.

Genes compose only part of the genome. The rest performs functions not involved with heredity. The exact number of human genes hasn't been determined with certainty. However, in its publication *A Guide to Your Genome*, the National Human Genome Research Institute estimated that humans have about 20,500 genes.

Hereditary Mutations and Acquired Mutations

The number of chromosomes an organism has differs among species. Humans have twenty-three pairs, a total of forty-six chromosomes.

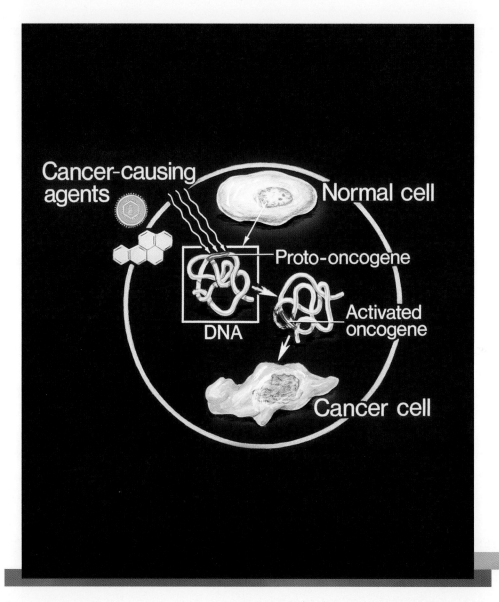

This diagram shows how a cancer-causing agent causes a proto-oncogene in a normal cell's DNA to mutate into an oncogene. This mutation transforms the cell into a cancer cell.

Each person inherits one set of twenty-three from his or her father and another set from his or her mother. Sometimes, genes on these chromosomes contain mutations. A genetic mutation is a change in a gene's DNA sequence. Because the sequence determines what protein a gene instructs the cell to make, any change can affect the cell's functioning. A mutation that a person inherits from a parent is called a hereditary mutation. It exists throughout a person's life and is present in all of the person's cells.

Genetic mutations can also be acquired. Environmental factors, such as smoking or the sun's rays, can damage DNA. Acquired mutations may also result from mistakes made when a cell is dividing. Acquired mutations aren't present in all of a person's cells and aren't usually passed on to a person's children.

Mutations and Cancer

Normal, healthy cells divide to form new cells only as the body needs them. Old or damaged cells die. Two types of genes that are important in this process play a role in cancer—proto-oncogenes and tumor suppressor genes.

Proto-oncogenes control how often a cell divides. When a proto-oncogene mutates into an oncogene, it can become permanently turned on. As a result, out-of-control cell growth occurs.

Tumor suppressor genes regulate the pace of cell division, repair errors in DNA, and tell cells when to die. When these genes don't work properly, the result is the same as when proto-oncogenes become oncogenes: the cell grows uncontrollably.

When cells with damaged DNA produce unneeded new cells or don't die as they should, there is out-of-control growth of abnormal cells. The usual consequence is a tumor—cancer. As the abnormal cells continue dividing, they may eventually invade other tissues.

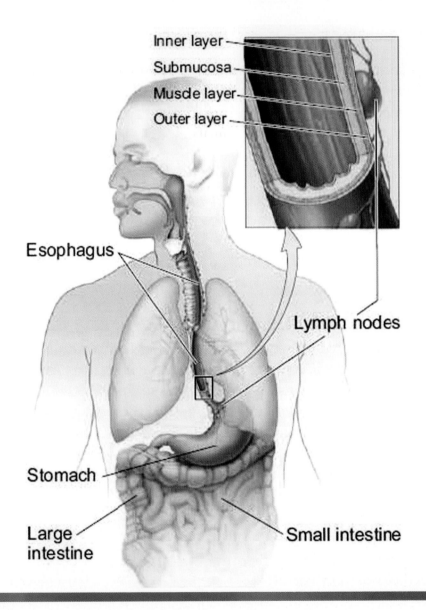

Inner layer
Submucosa
Muscle layer
Outer layer

Esophagus

Lymph nodes

Stomach

Large
intestine

Small intestine

This illustration shows the position of the esophagus within the body. The inset reveals the esophagus's four main layers. Lymph nodes surrounding the esophagus appear in green.

The Esophagus and Cancer

The esophagus is the hollow, muscular tube that connects the throat and stomach. Its function is to carry food and liquid from the mouth to the stomach.

The Structure of the Esophagus

The esophagus is usually 10 to 13 inches (25 to 33 centimeters) long. Its wall contains several layers. The innermost layer, the mucosa, is composed of two tissues. The epithelium lines the inside of the esophagus. It's composed of flat, thin squamous cells. Under the epithelium is the lamina propria, which is connective tissue.

The next layer is the submucosa. It contains mucus-secreting glands. Then comes a thick muscle layer called the muscularis propria. It pushes food along with peristalsis—coordinated, rhythmic muscle contractions. Enclosing all of these layers is the adventitia, a layer of connective tissue.

Two sphincters work with the muscularis propria to control the movement of food through the esophagus. The upper esophageal sphincter (UES) is a muscle at the top of the esophagus; the lower esophageal sphincter (LES) is a muscle at the bottom. When the UES relaxes, food and liquid can enter the esophagus. When the LES relaxes, food and liquid can move from the esophagus to the stomach.

Barrett's Esophagus and Changes in the Epithelium

In the condition known as Barrett's esophagus, the esophageal epithelium is transformed. Barrett's esophagus results from gastroesophageal reflux disease (GERD). In GERD, acid escapes from the stomach into the lower esophagus, often causing the burning sensation behind the lower end of the sternum (breastbone) that is called heartburn. Reflux can happen if the lower esophageal sphincter doesn't close well.

NORMAN BARRETT

How did Barrett's esophagus get its name? It was named for British surgeon Norman Barrett (1903–1979). Barrett specialized in the new field of thoracic, or chest, surgery. He was a brilliant surgeon and teacher who made many important contributions to the field. Today, he's chiefly remembered for his achievements in esophageal surgery. He published many articles on esophageal conditions, and, in a 1950 article, described a lower esophagus lined by columnar cells instead of normal epithelial ones.

Long-term GERD can have serious consequences. Acid in the stomach is normal and is important in the digestive process. It doesn't harm the cells lining the stomach because they're resistant to the acid. However, the acid can damage the lining of the lower esophagus, causing the squamous cells to be replaced with glandular cells. Unlike flat, thin squamous cells, glandular cells are columnar in shape. They're similar to the cells lining the stomach, and, like stomach cells, they release acid, enzymes, and mucus.

Esophageal Cancer

Both forms of esophageal cancer, squamous cell carcinoma and adenocarcinoma, start with mutations in mucosal cells. As the tumor grows, it expands outward through the other esophageal layers. Squamous cell carcinoma starts in epithelial squamous cells and can occur anywhere along the full length of the esophagus. However, adenocarcinoma only starts in glandular cells. Such cells aren't normally found in the esophagus.

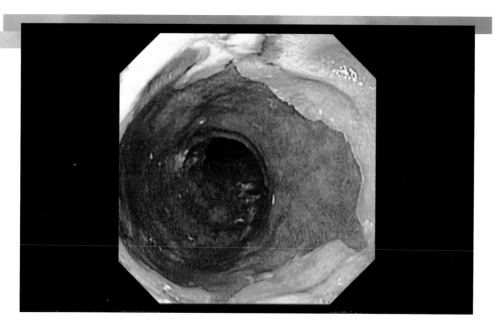

Barrett's esophagus is visible in this endoscopic image of an elderly male patient's lower esophagus. The red area contains Barrett's tissue. The pink area is the normal esophageal lining.

They only occur when Barrett's esophagus has transformed the lower esophageal lining. Thus, adenocarcinoma only develops when Barrett's esophagus already exists.

Over time, as esophageal cancer grows, it can invade nearby tissues. It can also metastasize, or spread to other parts of the body farther away. How is this possible? Cancer cells may break away from the original tumor, enter blood vessels or the lymph system, and be carried to other parts of the body. There, they may attach to tissue and form new tumors.

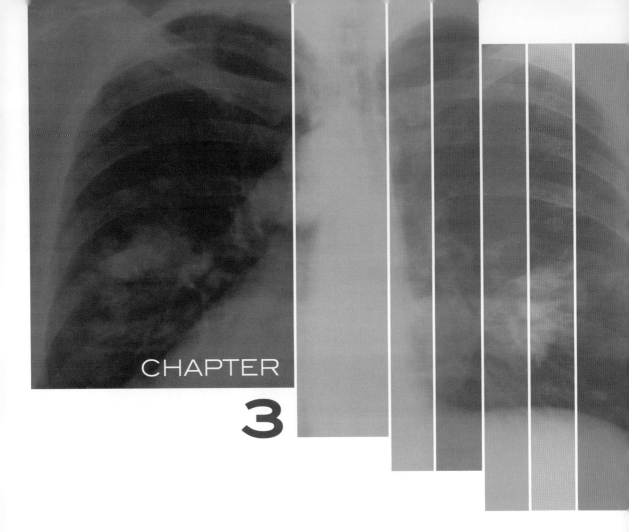

CHAPTER

3

WHO GETS ESOPHAGEAL CANCER, AND CAN IT BE PREVENTED?

In the United States, the risk of esophageal cancer is 1 in 200 (meaning that one out of every two hundred people will get esophageal cancer in his or her lifetime) according to *Esophageal Cancer*. In its publication *Cancer Facts & Figures 2010*, the ACS estimated about 16,640 new cases of esophageal cancer for 2010 and 14,500 deaths. For reasons that physicians don't understand, esophageal cancer rates are ten to one hundred times higher in Iran, northern China, India, and southern Africa. Differences also exist regarding what type of esophageal cancer is most common. In most of the world, squamous cell carcinoma occurs most often. In the United States, adenocarcinoma is most common.

The exact cause of esophageal cancer isn't known. However, researchers have identified certain risk factors for the disease.

Risk Factors

A risk factor is anything that may increase an individual's risk of a disease. Below are the major risk factors for esophageal cancer. Nonetheless, it's important to remember that having risk factors doesn't mean an individual will definitely develop the disease. Most people with risk factors don't develop esophageal cancer.

Age and Sex

The risk of esophageal cancer increases with age. Most cases in the United States occur in people who are sixty-five and older. Being male also increases risk. In the United States, men are three times more likely than women to be stricken.

Hereditary Conditions

Two inherited diseases—achalasia and tylosis—are risk factors for esophageal cancer. Fortunately, both conditions are rare.

Achalasia affects how well the esophagus functions. In this condition, peristalsis doesn't work well, and the lower esophageal sphincter does not relax properly. As a result, food and liquid don't move through the esophagus correctly and aren't able to pass into the stomach. They collect in the lower esophagus, which causes it to expand and damages its cells, thereby raising the risk of squamous cell carcinoma. In *Esophageal Cancer*, the ACS states that an achalasia patient has fifteen times the normal risk of developing esophageal cancer.

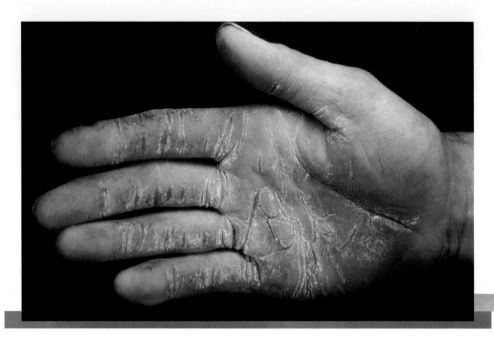

The thick, rough, grayish skin covering the palm of this person's hand indicates that the individual suffers from tylosis. This rare hereditary disease greatly increases the risk of developing esophageal cancer.

Tylosis is an extremely rare disease that causes excess growth of the top skin layer on the palms of the hands and soles of the feet. Sufferers also develop abnormal areas inside the mouth. The disease puts individuals at very high risk of squamous cell carcinoma.

RISKY BEHAVIORS

Researchers have identified several behaviors as risk factors. Most have long been linked to other cancers and health problems.

Cigarettes, cigars, pipes, and chewing tobacco increase an individual's risk. Both the amount that's used and how long it's used affect the risk. Tobacco products increase the risk of both forms of esophageal cancer.

Drinking alcoholic beverages increases the risk of squamous cell carcinoma. The more a person drinks, the greater the risk. Combining alcohol with tobacco use increases the risk much more than using either alone.

Diet affects an individual's risk. Overeating that results in obesity increases the risk of adenocarcinoma. A diet low in fruits and vegetables raises the risk. There's some evidence that processed meats, such as hot dogs, bologna, and sausage, may increase risk. Perhaps surprisingly, there's

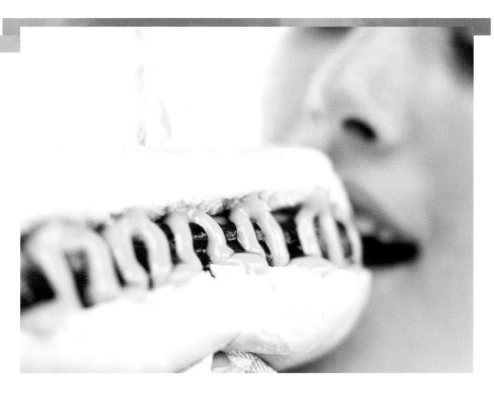

Hot dogs are enormously popular in the United States. They're standard fare at sporting events, amusement parks, and summer cookouts. Unfortunately, eating hot dogs may also increase a person's risk of developing esophageal cancer.

also evidence that frequently drinking liquids that are a very high temperature may raise the risk of squamous cell carcinoma.

OTHER RISK FACTORS

Numerous other risk factors have also been identified. Perhaps the most important is Barrett's esophagus, which, as described in chapter 2, involves the actual transformation of epithelial cells in the lower esophagus. In *Esophageal Cancer*, the ACS states that people with Barrett's esophagus are 30 to 125 times more likely to develop adenocarcinoma than people without it.

A related risk factor is GERD. One common cause of GERD is hiatal hernia. In this condition, part of the stomach sticks up into the chest cavity through the opening for the esophagus in the diaphragm (the band of muscle and connective tissue separating the chest and abdominal cavities). Pregnancy, obesity, cigarettes, alcohol, and some medications may also cause GERD.

Yet another risk factor related to both Barrett's esophagus and GERD is the eating disorder bulimia nervosa, often simply called bulimia. Individuals with this disorder are very unhappy with the way that their body looks and have an unreasonable fear of gaining weight. To avoid weight gain, they may take extreme measures such as making themselves vomit after eating to get rid of the food. Frequent vomiting subjects the esophagus to continuous acid erosion just as GERD does and may have the same consequences—that is, it may lead to Barrett's esophagus. There have been documented cases of people with a history of bulimia nervosa who have developed esophageal adenocarcinoma at a young age.

Some chemicals are risk factors. These include fumes from dry-cleaning and other chemicals. Lye, a harsh chemical compound used in some industrial and household cleaners, is another. Very young children

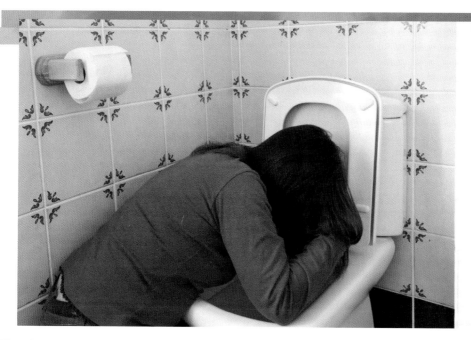

The frequent vomiting that often accompanies bulimia nervosa repeatedly subjects the esophagus to stomach acid and may lead to esophageal adenocarcinoma. The disorder is more common in women than men.

sometimes find cleaning products that aren't stored safely, and because they think these liquids are like milk or juice, they drink them. These cleaning liquids can burn the esophagus, resulting in scar tissue. People with such injuries have a high rate of squamous cell carcinoma as adults.

Esophageal webs raise the risk of squamous cell carcinoma. These abnormal bulges of tissue cause narrowing in the esophagus. People with webs usually have problems such as anemia, tongue irritation, brittle fingernails, and a large spleen.

People who've had lung, mouth, or throat cancer are at high risk of having esophageal cancer. This may be because all of these diseases are caused by smoking.

PREVENTION

Just as having risk factors doesn't guarantee a person will develop cancer, no actions can guarantee a person won't get cancer. However, a person can take steps to significantly reduce the risk of getting esophageal cancer.

One can't control one's age, whether one was born male or female, or the genes one inherited. However, one can control risky behaviors. A person can choose not to smoke (or to quit smoking if he or she has already started) and not to drink alcoholic beverages heavily. A person can choose to maintain a healthy diet, with plenty of fresh fruits and vegetables, and maintain a healthy weight by avoiding overeating and by exercising regularly.

Individuals who are suffering from heartburn or GERD should see a doctor to get treatment. People with GERD or Barrett's esophagus should have regular checkups so that their doctor can watch for early signs of esophageal cancer and begin treatment promptly. So how exactly do physicians diagnose and treat esophageal cancer? That's the topic of the next chapter.

MYTHS AND FACTS

MYTH **Heartburn is a minor problem, and smoking a cigarette can relieve the discomfort it causes.**

FACT Although common, heartburn isn't minor. It can be a symptom of GERD. Untreated, it can lead to esophagitis, Barrett's esophagus, and esophageal cancer. Far from relieving the discomfort, cigarette smoking may actually contribute to heartburn and GERD. Smokers suffer esophagitis that's probably caused by acid reflux. It's believed that cigarette smoking causes the LES to relax, allowing stomach acid to splash into the esophagus.

MYTH **Cigars are safer than cigarettes and thus less likely to cause esophageal cancer.**

FACT Cigars are just as dangerous as cigarettes. They're made of tobacco just like cigarettes and contain all the same dangerous chemicals. A large cigar may actually contain almost as much tobacco as a pack of cigarettes.

MYTH **Drinking soda causes esophageal adenocarcinoma.**

FACT Research published in the *Journal of the National Cancer Institute* in 2006 showed no link. However, drinking large amounts of sugary soft drinks can contribute to obesity, one of the risk factors for esophageal cancer.

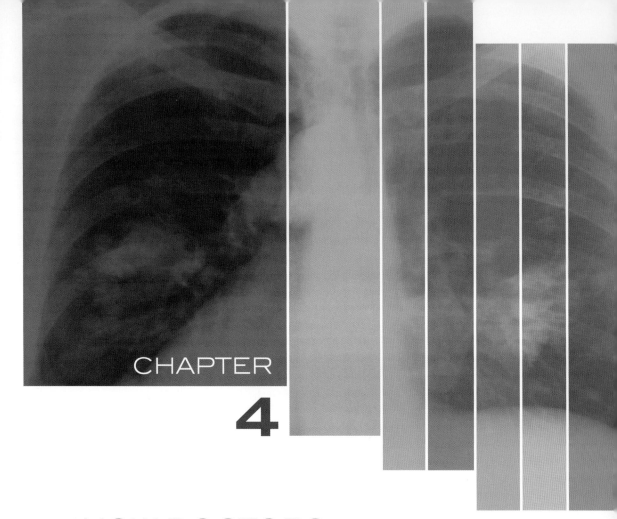

CHAPTER

4

HOW DOCTORS DIAGNOSE AND TREAT ESOPHAGEAL CANCER

The best chance of curing any cancer depends on discovering it early. Screening—testing or examining people for the presence of a disease—is designed to do that. However, there's no simple screening test for esophageal cancer. Because it usually doesn't cause symptoms in the early stages, it's generally discovered accidentally, as a result of tests done for other problems. More advanced esophageal cancer often displays symptoms such as the following:

- Difficulty swallowing (dysphagia)
- Pain when swallowing, or pain in the chest or back
- Weight loss
- Heartburn
- Hoarse voice or a cough that lasts longer than two weeks
- Other symptoms: hiccups, pneumonia, and high levels of calcium in the blood

A person who experiences these symptoms should see his or her doctor. The doctor can perform diagnostic tests and, if it's esophageal cancer, determine how advanced it is.

DIAGNOSING AND STAGING ESOPHAGEAL CANCER

First, the doctor gathers information on the patient's symptoms and past or present illnesses, medical conditions, and surgeries. A physical exam follows. Then, the doctor performs diagnostic tests.

DIAGNOSING ESOPHAGEAL CANCER

Often, the first test is a barium swallow, or upper GI series. The patient drinks a thick liquid called barium, then has X-rays taken. The barium coats the esophageal lining so that it stands out in the X-rays. Even small, early tumors show up clearly.

Another diagnostic test is an endoscopy (also called an upper endoscopy, EGD, or esophagoscopy). With an endoscope, the doctor examines the patient's esophageal lining for abnormal areas.

If an abnormal area is found, the doctor takes a small tissue sample for a biopsy, which is the only sure way to diagnose cancer. A physician called a pathologist examines the tissue under a microscope. If cancer cells are present, the pathologist determines whether they're squamous cell carcinoma or adenocarcinoma. Staging the cancer is next.

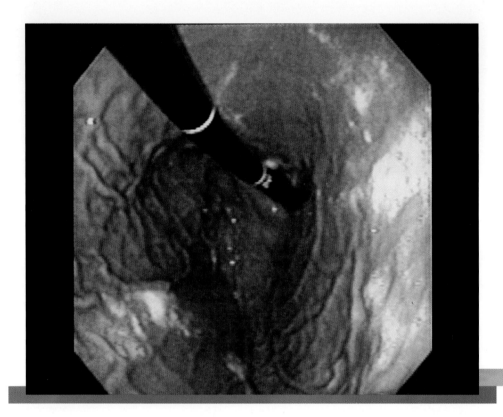

Endoscopies allow physicians remarkable views of the insides of living organs. In this image, the endoscope can be seen entering the stomach from the esophagus. The lining of this stomach is normal.

STAGES OF ESOPHAGEAL CANCER

Staging is the process of finding out the extent of the cancer. Esophageal cancer has five main stages. In Stage 0, abnormal cells only occur in the epithelium. Stage I cancer has reached the second layer, the submucosa. Stage II describes one of three conditions in which the cancer has spread beyond the submucosa: (1) cancer cells are in the lymph nodes, (2) the tumor has reached the muscularis propria, or (3) the cancer has reached the adventitia (the outermost layer). In Stage III, the tumor has grown through the adventitia and cancer cells are in the lymph nodes, or the cancer has invaded nearby structures (such as the airways). In Stage IV, cancer cells have spread to distant organs.

Staging Tests

How do doctors determine the stage? They conduct more tests.

Endoscopic ultrasound can be used to determine how deeply the tumor has invaded the esophageal wall. A probe at the end of an endoscope generates sound waves that bounce off the layers of the esophagus, and a computer uses the echoes to create a picture. An endoscope (without ultrasound) can also be used to visually examine the airways and the chest and abdominal cavities to see if cancer has spread to those regions.

Several imaging machines can show the cancer's spread. An X-ray machine linked to a computer takes CT scans, which are a series of detailed pictures. Magnetic resonance imaging (MRI) employs a strong magnet linked to a computer to take detailed pictures. PET scans and bone scans utilize machines that create images by tracking radioactive substances inserted into the body.

Treating Esophageal Cancer

After esophageal cancer has been diagnosed and staged, treatment follows. There are four main types of treatment—surgery, radiation therapy, chemotherapy, and endoscopic treatments. All have risks and side effects.

Surgery

Surgery to remove all or part of the esophagus, plus nearby lymph nodes, is called an esophagectomy. The upper part of the esophagus is then connected to the stomach. An esophagectomy may cure early-stage

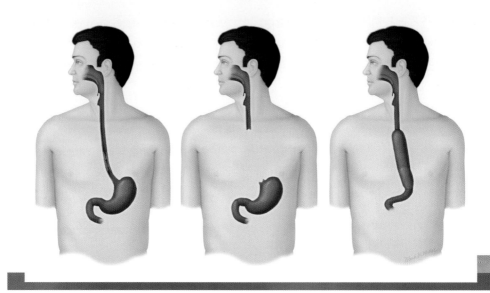

These illustrations show the stages of an esophagectomy: (1) normal positions of esophagus and stomach; (2) after removal of esophagus; and (3) stomach attached to upper part of esophagus.

cancer. In late-stage cancer, it can relieve symptoms, such as difficulty swallowing. There are, however, risks.

As with all serious surgeries, there's risk of a heart attack, a blood clot in the lungs or brain, or infection. Several problems specific to esophagectomies may arise following surgery. A leak may occur where the stomach and esophagus are connected; the stomach may empty too slowly, causing nausea and vomiting; narrowing where the stomach and esophagus are joined may cause problems swallowing; and removal of the LES may cause heartburn.

RADIATION THERAPY

Radiation therapy (radiotherapy) kills cancer cells with high-energy radiation. External beam radiation therapy, in which a machine outside the patient's body aims radiation at the cancer, is the most common for esophageal cancer. Internal radiation therapy (brachytherapy) puts radioactive material directly into or near the cancer. Radiation therapy may be used alone, but it's usually combined with surgery or chemotherapy. It may also be used for palliative therapy, or relief of symptoms caused by a large cancerous mass.

Radiation therapy has several side effects. Skin in the treated area may seem sunburned or develop blisters or open sores. There may be hair loss. Painful sores may develop in the mouth and throat. The patient may experience nausea, vomiting, and diarrhea. Fatigue is common in the later stages of treatment. Sometimes, the radiation damages healthy esophageal tissue, resulting in painful swallowing.

CHEMOTHERAPY

In chemotherapy (chemo), the patient receives powerful drugs through a vein or by mouth. Common chemotherapy drugs include 5-fluorouracil (5-FU), capecitibine, cisplatin, carboplatin, oxaloplatin, doxorubicin, and epirubicin. Because the drugs travel through the bloodstream and reach all parts of the body, this therapy is useful to treat both the primary cancer and any metastases (cells that have spread to other places in the body). Chemotherapy is rarely used alone. It may be given before surgery to shrink the tumor or after surgery to kill any remaining cancer cells. It's often combined with radiation therapy (chemoradiation or chemoradiotherapy). Like radiation, chemotherapy can be used for palliative therapy to decrease symptoms of the cancer or prolong a person's life, even though the cancer isn't curable.

Chemotherapy's general side effects result from its effects on normal cells that also divide rapidly. These include blood cells, cells in hair roots, and cells that line digestive system organs. Common side effects are nausea and vomiting, diarrhea, mouth sores, loss of appetite, hair loss, fatigue, increased risk of infection, problems with bleeding or bruising, and skin rash.

ENDOSCOPIC TREATMENTS

Endoscopic treatments are mostly used to treat dysplasia (precancer) and very early cancers or to relieve swallowing problems. With the aid of an endoscope, the physician applies instruments, lasers, high-power energy, and even electric current to problem areas.

CLINICAL TRIALS

A clinical trial is a carefully controlled study done with patients who volunteer. Trials are done to test promising new drugs, treatments, or procedures. Patients interested in participating must meet certain requirements. Those who don't meet the conditions won't be accepted. Trials usually follow years of research and animal testing, and they offer patients access to state-of-the-art treatments that they couldn't get otherwise. Nonetheless, clinical trials are not without some risk, and patients may or may not benefit from the new therapy in comparison to the existing standard of care. The hope of a clinical trial is to find an even better treatment than what is currently available.

COMPLEMENTARY AND ALTERNATIVE THERAPIES

Complementary and alternative therapies are treatments outside the standard medical therapies. Various people use these terms differently. Here, "complementary" refers to treatments used *in addition to* regular medical care. "Alternative" refers to treatments used *instead of* standard medical therapy.

Typically, complementary therapies are used to help a patient feel better and deal with the diseases and treatments. These therapies include meditation, acupuncture, massage, herbal teas, and aromatherapy.

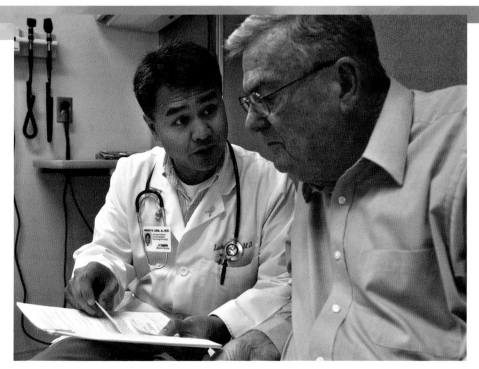

Clinical trials are essential to the development of new drugs, treatments, and procedures to treat diseases. Here, a doctor encourages a cancer patient to take part in a clinical trial.

Meditation consists of mental exercises designed to create a state of peace and relaxation. Acupuncture is an ancient Chinese practice in which thin needles are inserted at specific points in the body to relieve pain and treat disease. Massage is a method of rubbing and kneading the body's muscle and soft tissue. Aromatherapy is the use of fragrant plant oils. Many people find that meditation and aromatherapy reduce the stress that accompanies a life-threatening illness. Some people find that acupuncture or massage relieves pain. Acupuncture, aromatherapy, and drinking peppermint tea reduce nausea for some people.

Alternative therapies may be presented as cancer cures. By their very nature, they have not undergone years of research and testing, and the U.S. Food and Drug Administration (FDA) does not regulate them. This means that neither their safety nor their effectiveness has been proven. Although some alternative therapies may provide some benefits, others may be dangerous or even life threatening. The extravagant and unproven claims sometimes presented for alternative therapies may induce patients diagnosed with a deadly illness to try them. When the promised results don't materialize, patients may return to standard medical treatment. However, by that time, the disease is more advanced and less likely to respond to any treatment. Anyone considering alternative therapy needs to gather as much information as possible and discuss options with his or her doctor.

TEN GREAT QUESTIONS TO ASK YOUR DOCTOR

1. What kind of esophageal cancer is it?

2. What stage is it?

3. Has the cancer spread?

4. What is the goal of treatment?

5. What are the treatment options?

6. Will more than one kind of treatment be administered?

7. Will a hospital stay be required?

8. What are the risks and possible side effects of each treatment?

9. Would a clinical trial be a good treatment choice?

10. Will more tests be needed during or after treatment?

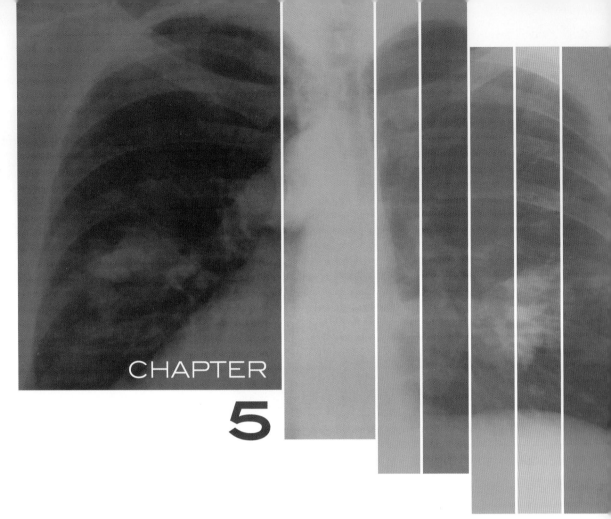

CHAPTER

5

DEALING WITH CANCER, TREATMENT, AND LIFE AFTERWARD

Both esophageal cancer and the treatment for it can cause other health problems. They're also emotionally challenging. This chapter addresses some of the problems and ways to deal with them.

DIFFICULTY SWALLOWING

As discussed in chapter 4, difficult or painful swallowing is a common symptom of esophageal cancer. It results from the tumor blocking the

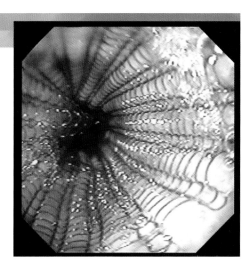

Seen through an endoscope, a metal stent opens a blockage in a patient's esophagus. It's easy to see how large chunks of food could get caught in the stent.

esophagus. It can cause patients to change their diet and thus can lead to poor nutrition. Fortunately, several forms of palliative therapy are available to treat this problem.

BALLOON DILATION

The physician inserts an endoscope down the esophagus to the blockage. A deflated balloon is passed through the endoscope and then inflated. The pressure widens the opening, making it easier for the patient to swallow. The physician removes the balloon immediately after the procedure.

ESOPHAGEAL STENTS

A stent is a tube of metal or plastic mesh. The physician gives the patient a drug to relax him or her, then inserts the stent into the blockage with an endoscope. The stent expands, creating an opening for the passage of food and liquid. Unlike the balloon, the stent remains in the esophagus. This means that, after the procedure, the patient must always chew solid foods thoroughly before swallowing to prevent food chunks from becoming stuck in the stent and causing a blockage.

Light Therapies

Two forms of light therapy may be used to remove blockages. One is called laser therapy or laser ablation. It involves using a laser's concentrated light beam to kill cancer cells.

The other form of light therapy is called photodynamic therapy. The patient first receives an injection of a drug, which is allowed to collect in the cancer cells for a few days. Then the physician uses an endoscope to shine a special type of laser light on the tumor. The light produces a change in the drug that makes it deadly to cancer cells, thus shrinking the blockage.

Heat Therapies

Two therapies use electric current to generate heat. In electrocoagulation, electric current is used to burn off tissue. In argon plasma coagulation (APC), electric current changes argon gas into a plasma that is used to burn the tumor.

Radiation Therapy and Chemotherapy

As discussed in chapter 4, radiation therapy and chemotherapy are both standard treatments for esophageal cancer. They're also used as palliative therapy to relieve problems with swallowing.

Pain Management

Pain often accompanies esophageal cancer, just as it does other cancers. It may also be a side effect of some treatments. Controlling pain is essential to helping the patient maintain the best quality of life possible. Numerous medications are available to treat pain in cancer patients. In addition, as mentioned in chapter 4, some patients find that complementary therapies like acupuncture and massage provide effective pain relief.

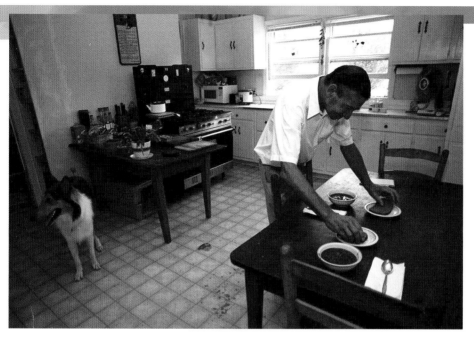

*Cancer patients sometimes face surprising challenges to good nutrition.
Radiation therapy for esophageal cancer caused this man to lose his teeth and
forced him to develop a diet suitable for denture wearers.*

NUTRITION

During treatment, problems with swallowing may lead to poor nutrition. Good nutrition can help the patient feel better and have more energy. Obviously, getting palliative therapy to improve swallowing is an important first step to good nutrition. However, other obstacles may present themselves. The patient may simply be too tired to eat. Chemotherapy can change the way foods taste. Treatment side effects such as poor appetite, nausea, vomiting, and diarrhea can cause a patient to not eat well. If any of these developments create problems with eating, the patient should meet with a registered dietitian. The dietitian may suggest changing the texture or the fat and fiber content of food to make swallowing easier. The dietitian may also suggest eating several small meals each day instead of three large meals. Sometimes, liquid meals may be a patient's best option. In the most difficult situations, it may be necessary to rely on a feeding tube or intravenous nutrition.

After treatment, the patient may need to make adjustments to his or her diet. This usually just means making an extra effort to follow the nutritional guidelines recommended for everyone. Eat five or more servings of fruits and vegetables daily, eat whole-grain foods, reduce the amount of fat in the diet, reduce or eliminate processed meats, limit alcohol consumption, and limit consumption of very sweet foods and drinks (such as sodas).

Following surgery, where removal of the esophagus and perhaps part of the stomach has radically altered the way the digestive system processes food, the patient may have problems with diarrhea, cramps, nausea, bloating, sweating, and dizziness. These are symptoms of what is called "dumping syndrome." After an esophagectomy, the stomach effectively replaces the esophagus and thus can't perform all of its former functions. The stomach can no longer hold food for digestion as it once did, and the food is "dumped" into the intestine too quickly. The patient can take several measures to help control dumping syndrome. Eating smaller meals and eating more often helps. So does drinking liquids before or after eating solid foods. Staying upright for several hours after eating may also help. Patients who have had surgery may need to take vitamin and mineral supplements daily, too.

There are several other steps the patient should take to maintain the best quality of life possible. A smoker should quit smoking. Exercise will make the patient feel better and give him or her more energy. It's important to keep all follow-up appointments with the doctor and report any new symptoms. The patient should also seek palliative treatment for any symptoms that cause problems.

WHEN TREATMENT DOESN'T WORK

Because esophageal cancer is usually caught late and thus is often fatal, patients and their families frequently find themselves facing the harsh reality that treatment isn't working. Overwhelming emotions compound the pain of physical suffering. Difficult choices must be made. Should the patient continue treatment if improvement is extremely unlikely? Should a very weak patient remain in the hospital or go home? Is hospice a good choice? Whatever decision is made, the patient should seek or continue palliative therapy to remain as comfortable as possible. Sources of support are especially important. Friends, religious leaders, and professional counselors can all provide support.

DEALING WITH EMOTIONS

Having a life-threatening illness such as cancer is one of the most difficult situations that an individual can face. It can also feel very lonely. It's important for the patient to talk about his or her feelings and experiences. Each patient should choose the sources of support that work best for him or her. Sources include family, friends, professional counselors, religious or spiritual groups, and support groups. If a patient wants to join a support group and doesn't know where to find one, the American Cancer Society and the National Cancer Institute (NCI) can help. Call the ACS at (800) 227-2345. Call the NCI at (800) 4-CANCER [(800) 422-6237]. A patient who cannot find a support group nearby or isn't physically able to go can participate in online support communities. Taking steps to care for one's emotional as well as physical health is an important element of dealing with cancer.

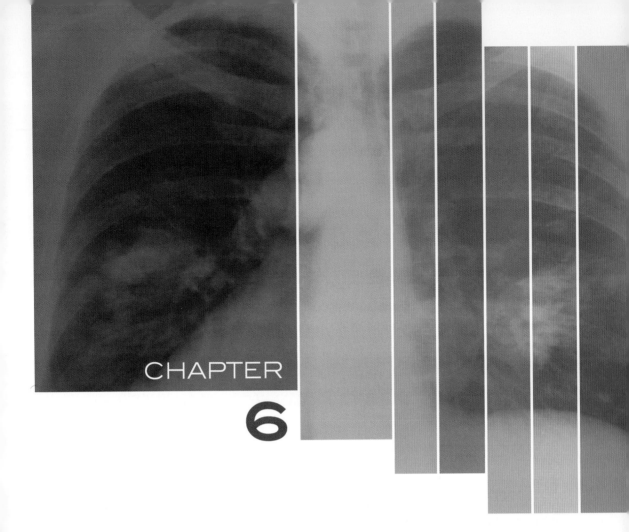

CHAPTER

6

DIRECTIONS IN ESOPHAGEAL CANCER RESEARCH AND TREATMENT

What does the future hold for esophageal cancer? What kind of research is currently being conducted on this deadly and increasingly common disease?

The early twenty-first century has seen an enormous amount of research into many aspects of esophageal cancer. Major areas of research include finding ways to predict who's likely to develop the disease, finding ways to prevent it, developing screening tests, and discovering new and more effective treatments.

Because of the link between Barrett's esophagus and esophageal adenocarcinoma, much of the research actually focuses on Barrett's esophagus rather than esophageal cancer itself. New drugs and new developments in technology figure prominently in recent research. So do genetic discoveries. These have been greatly advanced by the completion of the Human Genome Project, which established the sequence of nucleotides in the entire human genome.

Predicting Who Will Develop Esophageal Cancer

Identifying the factors that make a person highly likely to develop esophageal cancer can improve monitoring and screening, hopefully leading to earlier diagnosis and improved survival rates. Much research is focusing on identifying genetic predictors of esophageal cancer. For example, in 2008, researchers at M. D. Anderson Cancer Center in Houston, Texas, announced that they had identified eleven genetic variations that could increase an individual's risk of developing esophageal cancer. In 2009, researchers at the University of Tokyo identified two genetic variations that increased the risk of esophageal cancer in Japanese people, especially when combined with alcohol and tobacco use.

Similar research is ongoing. Researchers at M. D. Anderson Cancer Center are trying to determine if certain biomarkers (genes and proteins) can predict whether an individual with Barrett's esophagus will actually go on to develop esophageal adenocarcinoma. Researchers at the Mayo Clinic, an acclaimed medical practice headquartered in Rochester, Minnesota, are looking for genes involved in the development of Barrett's esophagus and esophageal cancer.

THE HUMAN GENOME PROJECT

The U.S. National Institutes of Health (NIH) and the U.S. Department of Energy (DOE), aided by international organizations, launched the Human Genome Project in 1990. The goal was to determine the sequence of the nucleotides in human DNA and identify all of the genes in the human genome. By 2003, researchers had established the nucleotide sequence of the entire human genome. They had mapped the locations of genes on all human chromosomes by 2006. The project's achievements greatly advanced research into the role of genetics in human disease. Here are some fascinating facts discovered by the Human Genome Project:

— The human genome contains about 2.85 billion nucleotides.

— The average gene contains three thousand nucleotides.

— Dystrophin, the largest gene, is responsible for the production of a muscle protein and contains about 2.4 million nucleotides.

— Chromosome 1, the largest chromosome, contains 3,141 genes.

PREVENTING ESOPHAGEAL CANCER

Some recent and ongoing research is seeking ways to prevent Barrett's esophagus from developing into esophageal adenocarcinoma. For example, a promising new therapy called HALO ablation is being used to treat Barrett's esophagus. This procedure uses a short burst of radio-frequency ablation to remove Barrett's tissue. Healthy tissue then grows in to replace the tissue that was removed. Unlike electrocoagulation and argon plasma coagulation, HALO ablation can be precisely controlled so that only the Barrett's tissue is removed, not healthy tissue. The treatment is also much simpler and less likely to produce serious side effects than esophagectomy.

Ongoing prevention studies include one at M. D. Anderson that's studying whether green tea extract can reduce the risk of Barrett's esophagus developing into adenocarcinoma. A study at the Mayo Clinic is comparing the effects of esomeprazole (a drug used to treat GERD) in people with Barrett's esophagus to the effects of esomeprazole combined with aspirin to see if they affect an individual's risk of developing esophageal cancer.

SCREENING

New techniques have recently been developed to screen for Barrett's esophagus. One of these is narrow band imaging (NBI), which uses colored light to examine the esophagus, rather than the traditional white light. NBI is based on the fact that different colors of light penetrate tissue to different depths depending on their wavelength. Blue light, which has a short wavelength, doesn't penetrate deeply. Red light, with its longer wavelength, does. NBI uses a red-green-blue sequence of light to create images of the esophageal lining. A computer then combines the three images to produce a much clearer and more detailed image that improves diagnosis.

Another recent screening method is esophageal capsule endoscopy. In this procedure, the patient swallows a tiny camera and transmitter. The camera takes pictures as it passes through the esophagus, and the transmitter sends them to a receiver. The images are then displayed on a screen for the physician. Capsule endoscopy was developed in the

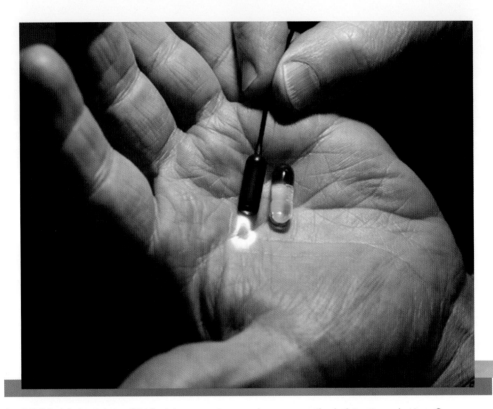

In 2008, University of Washington researchers unveiled this tiny device for detecting esophageal cancer. It's roughly the size of an ordinary capsule and contains a miniature laser scanner.

1990s and can be used to take pictures anywhere in the gastrointestinal tract. It was approved for use in the esophagus in 2004.

TREATMENT

In the area of esophageal cancer treatment, an immense amount of recent and ongoing research focuses on chemotherapy. Some of the research examines the effects of single drugs. More often, the research focuses on combinations of drugs or on combined therapies involving drugs and radiation therapy or surgery. One new and exciting area of chemotherapy research deals with targeted cancer therapies.

Unlike the treatments discussed in chapter 4, targeted cancer therapies actually work at the molecular level. These drugs block the growth of cancer by interfering with the specific molecules involved in tumor growth. Most target therapies are small molecule drugs or monoclonal antibodies. "What on Earth are those?" the reader may be asking. Well, small molecule drugs are able to bind to or pass through the membrane surrounding a cell to act on targets within the cell. Monoclonal antibodies usually can't pass through the cell membrane. They act on targets outside of the cell or on the cell surface.

Some target therapies block the specific enzymes and growth factor receptors involved in the multiplication of cancer cells. Others block angiogenesis, which is the growth of blood vessels to tumors. Still others help the immune system destroy cancer cells. Some monoclonal antibodies are actually used to deliver toxic molecules directly to the cancer cells!

Another emerging approach to treating esophageal cancer is gene therapy. This involves correcting mutated genes responsible for disease development. Usually, this means inserting a normal gene into the genome to replace an abnormal gene. Gene therapy was first used in 1990 but is still experimental. It's incredibly difficult and has been attempted in human trials only a few times. In some trials, it's failed to correct the disease being treated or even caused other diseases. Occasionally, it's resulted in deaths. No gene therapies currently exist for esophageal cancer. However, there's hope that growing knowledge of the genetic changes apparently associated with esophageal cancer will lead to gene therapies for the disease. In fact, researchers in Japan are continuing gene therapy research that was begun around 2000. Their research focuses on correcting a tumor suppressor gene that frequently shows mutations in esophageal cancer.

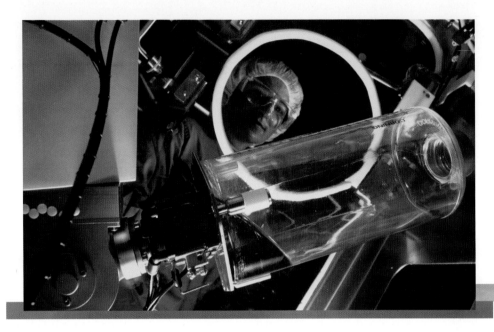

This laboratory technician uses robotic machinery to create monoclonal antibodies. These antibodies are all genetically identical because they're all copies of the same original cell. They all recognize the same substance.

For the present, esophageal cancer remains a difficult disease to treat. Still, the growth in its occurrence has helped prompt increased research. The emergence of new drugs, development of technologies that permit targeted therapies, and advancement in knowledge about human genes have opened whole new areas of research. Researchers are aggressively pursuing many paths. There's reason to hope that esophageal cancer will become a more treatable disease in the future.

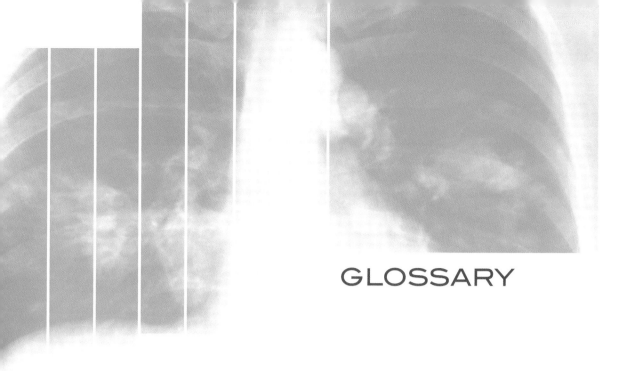

GLOSSARY

ablation The process of removing by cutting or evaporating.

anemia A condition in which the blood lacks sufficient red blood cells; there are many types of anemia and many underlying causes.

barium A soft, silver-white metal; a mixture of barium sulfate and water, opaque to X-rays, that a patient swallows to permit radiological examination of the digestive tract.

benign Not life threatening; harmless in effect.

biopsy The removal and examination of tissue from a living body.

connective tissue A kind of body tissue that supports and binds other tissues together.

contraction The shortening and thickening of a working muscle.

diagnose To identify a disease.

endoscopy The examination of a hollow organ, such as the esophagus, with an endoscope.

enzyme A type of complex protein produced by living cells.

heredity The passing on of characteristics from one generation to the next through genes.

hospice A type of medical care designed to promote the comfort of terminally ill patients; hospice care may be given in a patient's home or in a special palliative facility.

lymph A pale liquid that circulates through the body and carries immune cells.

malignant A cancerous tumor that can spread to other organs; liable to cause death.

obesity A condition characterized by excessive body fat.

palliative Relating to the easing of symptoms without curing the underlying disease.

plasma A collection of charged particles that exhibits some properties of a gas but is a good conductor of electricity.

radioactive Spontaneously emitting charged particles.

risk factor Anything that makes it more likely a person will develop a disease.

sphincter A circular muscle that surrounds a body opening and can close the opening.

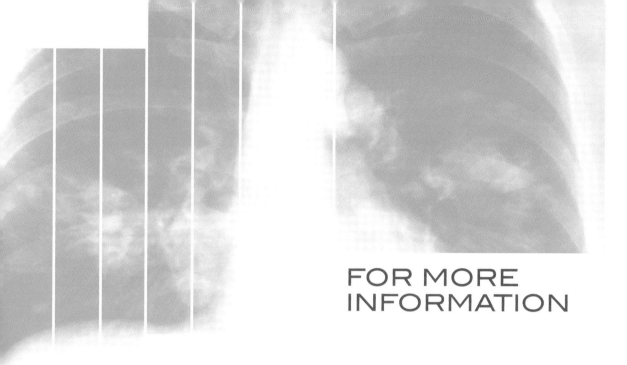

FOR MORE INFORMATION

American Cancer Society (ACS)
250 Williams Street
Atlanta, GA 30303
(800) ACS-2345 [(800) 227-2345]
Web site: http://www.cancer.org
The ACS is the nationwide health organization dedicated to preventing cancer, saving lives, and diminishing suffering from cancer through research, education, advocacy, and service.

American Institute for Cancer Research (AICR)
1759 R Street NW
Washington, DC 20009
(800) 843-8114; (202) 328-7744 in DC
Web site: http://www.aicr.org
The AICR funds research on the relationship of nutrition, physical activity, and weight management to cancer risk; interprets scientific literature on cancer; and educates people about choices they can make to reduce their chances of developing cancer.

Canadian Cancer Society
National Office
10 Alcorn Avenue, Suite 200
Toronto, ON M4V 3B1
Canada
(416) 961-7223
Web site: http://www.cancer.ca
The Canadian Cancer Society is a national, community-based organization of volunteers dedicated to the eradication of cancer and the enhancement of the quality of life of people living with cancer.

Canadian Digestive Health Foundation (CDHF)
1500 Upper Middle Road, Unit 3
P.O. Box 76059
Oakville, ON L6M 3H5
Canada
(905) 829-3949
Web site: http://www.cdhf.ca
The CDHF is the foundation of the Canadian Association of Gastroenterology. Its mission is to reduce suffering and improve quality of life by providing trusted, accessible, and accurate information about digestive health and diseases.

Esophageal Cancer Awareness Association
P.O. Box 55071 #15530
Boston, MA 02205-5071
(800) 601-0613
Web site: http://www.ecaware.org
Established in 2002, the Esophageal Cancer Awareness Association works to help esophageal cancer patients, survivors, and their

caregivers deal more effectively with the uncertainties of this disease and its consequences.

National Cancer Institute (NCI)
NCI Public Inquiries Office
6116 Executive Boulevard, Room 3036A
Bethesda, MD 20892-8322
(800) 422-6237
Web site: http://www.cancer.gov
The NCI is part of the National Institutes of Health. Established under the National Cancer Institute Act of 1937, it is the federal government's principal agency for cancer research and training.

WEB SITES

Due to the changing nature of Internet links, Rosen Publishing has developed an online list of Web sites related to the subject of this book. This site is updated regularly. Please use this link to access the list:

http://www.rosenlinks.com/cms/eso

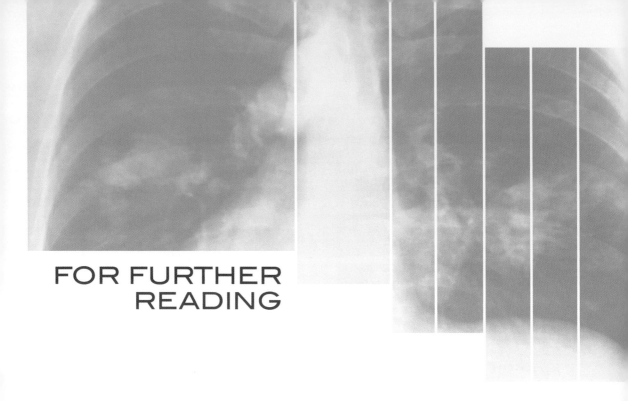

FOR FURTHER READING

Berman, Jules J. *Precancer: The Beginning and the End of Cancer.* Sudbury, MA: Jones and Bartlett Publishers, 2010.

Burns, David L., and Neeral L. Shah. *100 Questions & Answers About Gastroesophageal Reflux Disease (GERD): A Lahey Clinic Guide.* Sudbury, MA: Jones and Bartlett Publishers, 2007.

Dreyer, ZoAnn. *Living with Cancer* (Teen's Guides). New York, NY: Checkmark Books, 2008.

Ginex, Pamela K., Maureen Jingeleski, Bart L. Frazzitta, and Manjit S. Bains. *100 Questions & Answers About Esophageal Cancer.* 2nd ed. Sudbury, MA: Jones and Bartlett Publishers, 2010.

Grant, Barbara, Abby S. Bloch, Kathryn K. Hamilton, and Cynthia A. Thomson. *American Cancer Society Complete Guide to Nutrition for Cancer Survivors: Eating Well, Staying Well During and After Cancer.* Atlanta, GA: American Cancer Society, 2010.

Henry, Julie. *Getting Answers About Cancer: Understanding the Symptoms, Diagnosis and Treatment.* San Clemente, CA: Shining Lion Publications, 2009.

Kornmehl, Carol. *The Best News About Radiation Therapy: Everything You Need to Know About Your Treatment*. Howell, NJ: Academic Radiation Oncology Press, 2003.

Kudla, Ronald J. *Planting the Roses: A Cancer Survivor's Story*. Cleveland, OH: Cleveland Clinic Press, 2005.

Lew, Kristi. *The Truth About Cancer: Understanding and Fighting a Deadly Disease* (Issues in Focus Today). Berkeley Heights, NJ: Enslow Publishers, 2009.

MacDonald, Gayle. *Medicine Hands: Massage Therapy for People with Cancer*. Forres, Scotland: Findhorn Press, 2007.

McKay, Judith, and Tamera Schacher. *The Chemotherapy Survival Guide: Everything You Need to Know to Get Through Treatment*. Oakland, CA: New Harbinger Publications, 2009.

Panno, Joseph. *Cancer* (New Biology). New York, NY: Facts On File, 2010.

Panno, Joseph. *Cancer: The Role of Genes, Lifestyle, and Environment* (New Biology). New York, NY: Facts On File, 2004.

Shah, Manish A. *Dx/Rx: Upper Gastrointestinal Malignancies: Cancers of the Stomach and Esophagus*. Sudbury, MA: Jones and Bartlett Publishers, 2005.

Turkington, Carol, and William Lipera. *The Encyclopedia of Cancer* (Facts On File Library of Health and Living). New York, NY: Facts On File, 2005.

Williams, Carl O., ed. *Cancer of the Esophagus: A Reference Guide and Bibliography*. Hauppage, NY: Nova Science Publishers, 2010.

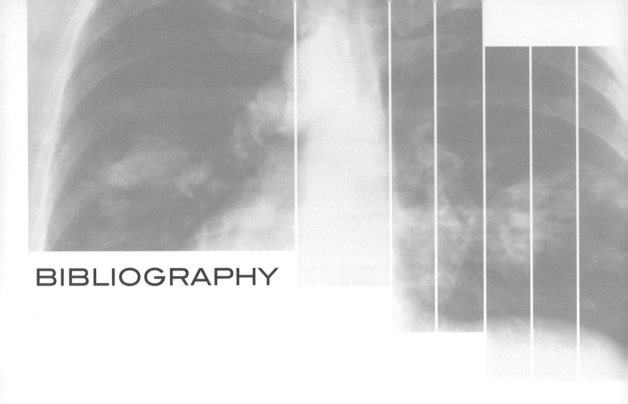

BIBLIOGRAPHY

American Cancer Society. *Cancer Facts & Figures 2010*. Atlanta, GA: American Cancer Society, 2010.

American Cancer Society. *Esophageal Cancer*. Atlanta, GA: American Cancer Society, 2009.

American Cancer Society. "Oncogenes and Tumor Suppressor Genes." Retrieved February 27, 2010 (http://www.cancer.org/docroot/ETO/content/ETO_1_4x_oncogenes_and_tumor_suppressor_genes.asp?sitearea=ETO&viewmode=print&).

American Cancer Society, Cancer Reference Information. "The History of Cancer." 2009. Retrieved January 10, 2010 (http://www.cancer.org/docroot/CRI/content/CRI_2_6x_the_history_of_cancer_72.asp?sitearea=CRI&viewmode=print&).

Eslick, Guy D. "Esophageal Cancer: A Historical Perspective." *Gastroenterology Clinics of North America*, Vol. 38, No. 1 (2009), pp. 1–15.

Human Genome Project Information. "Gene Therapy." Oak Ridge National Laboratory. Retrieved March 14, 2010 (http://www.ornl.gov/sci/techresources/Human_Genome/medicine/genetherapy.shtml).

Lord, Reginald V. N. "Norman Barrett, 'Doyen of Esophageal Surgery.'" *Annals of Surgery*, Vol. 229, No. 3 (1999), pp. 428–439.

Mayne, Susan T., et al. "Carbonated Soft Drink Consumption and Risk of Esophageal Adenocarcinoma." *Journal of the National Cancer Institute*, Vol. 98, No. 1 (January 4, 2006), pp. 72–75.

National Cancer Institute. "Esophageal Cancer Prevention, Patient Version." 2007. Retrieved January 8, 2010 (http://www.cancer.gov/cancertopics/pdq/prevention/esophageal/patient).

National Cancer Institute. "Esophageal Cancer Screening, Patient Version." 2007. Retrieved January 8, 2010 (http://www.cancer.gov/cancertopics/pdq/screening/esophageal/patient).

National Cancer Institute. "Esophageal Cancer Treatment, Patient Version." 2007. Retrieved January 8, 2010 (http://www.cancer.gov/cancertopics/pdq/treatment/esophageal/patient).

National Cancer Institute. "Targeted Cancer Therapies." Factsheet. Retrieved February 19, 2010 (http://www.cancer.gov/cancertopics/factsheet/Therapy/targeted).

National Cancer Institute. *What You Need to Know About Cancer of the Esophagus*. Bethesda, MD: National Cancer Institute, n.d.

National Cancer Institute, Office of Science Planning and Assessment. "A Snapshot of Esophageal Cancer." Bethesda, MD: National Cancer Institute, 2008.

National Human Genome Research Institute. *A Guide to Your Genome*. Bethesda, MD: National Institutes of Health, 2007.

Shimada, Hideaki, Kazuyuki Matsushita, and Masatoshi Tagawa. "Recent Advances in Esophageal Cancer Gene Therapy." *Annals of Thoracic Cardiovascular Surgery*, Vol. 14, No. 1 (2008), pp. 3–8.

Shinohara, Eric T., et al. "Esophageal Cancer in a Young Woman with Bulimia Nervosa: A Case Report." *Journal of Medical Case Reports*, Vol. 1, No. 160 (November 29, 2007).

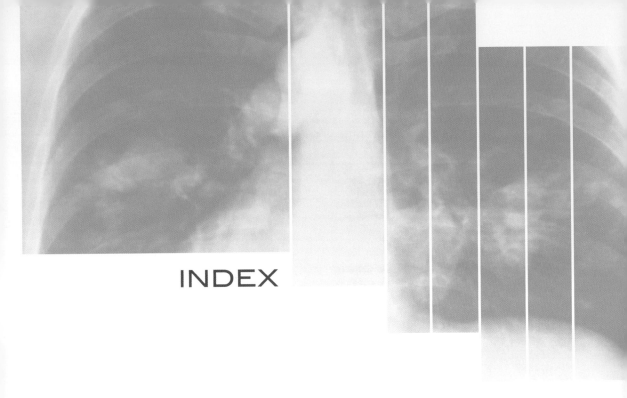

INDEX

ABOUT THE AUTHOR

Janey Levy is a writer and editor who lives in Colden, New York. She's the author of more than one hundred books for children and young adults. Levy has written on a variety of science topics, including genetic diseases, elements of the periodic table, conservation, and biomes and habitats. Her interest in cancer stems from the fact that several members of her family have had various forms of the disease. She also has a friend whose uncle died from esophageal cancer.

PHOTO CREDITS

Cover, p. 1 © Alan Hinerfeld/CMSP; cover (top), pp. 4–5 (bottom) Punchstock; back cover, pp. 3, 7, 14, 16, 18, 22, 30, 40, 46, 53, 55, 58, 60, 62 National Cancer Institute; p. 8 http://ihm.nlm.nih.gov; p. 11 © SSPL/The Image Works; p. 13 Courtesy of the University of Alabama at Birmingham; p. 21 © Science Photo Library/CMSP; p. 24 © NMSB/CMSP; p. 25 Stockbyte/Thinkstock; p. 27 © www.istockphoto.com/ jean gill; p. 32 © S. Benjamin/CMSP; p. 34 © Mark Miller/Photo Researchers, Inc.; p. 37 © Jay Mather/Sacramento Bee/ZUMA Press; p. 41 © David M. Martin, M.D./ Photo Researchers, Inc.; p. 43 © AP Images; p. 50 Dean Rutz/Seattle Times/ MCT/Newscom; p. 52 © James King-Holmes/Automation Partnership/Photo Researchers, Inc.

Designer: Evelyn Horowicz; Editor: Kathy Kuhtz Campbell;
Photo Researcher: Amy Feinberg